Senior-Cize

CHAIR YOGA EDITION

Gentle Exercises for Flexibility, Strength, and Peace of Mind

By Tony R. Wright

CONTENTS

DEDICATION TO PARENTS

"To my mother and father,who never stopped believing in me."
Thanks for keeping the interest rates low on everything I owe you." (Remember When!)

INTRODUCTION

Fitness is crucial for Senior Citizens since, their bones become more brittle as they age. If Senior citizens become sedimentary, they are more liable to break a bone versesyoung healthy individual. There are many reasons why we tend to slow down and sit longer as we age. It may be due to health issues, weight or pain issues, or fear of falling. Or, you might think that exercise is not for you at all. But as you get older, an active lifestyle is more important to your health than ever. **Senior-Cize** enables our seniors to perform low impact movements that still connects them to a healthy lifestyle.

Benefits of Senior-Cize:

- **Reduce Joint Pain in Just 10 Min a Day:** Step-by-Step progressions with a 4-week plan to feel at your best!
- **Fight Aging with Gentle Routines:** Exercises and Workouts designed by a Personal Trainer + 5 Motivational Cues for Seniors to stay on track of your fitness journey!
- **Feel Stronger Just After a Few Days:** Learn easy-to-follow Illustrated exercises for Stretching, Toning and feeling stronger to enhance your sense of well-being.
- **Improve Balance and Avoid Risk of Falling:** Illustrated Step-by-Step Guide designed by a Personal Trainer to perform the exercise safely and effective.
- **Boost Your Energy Levels:** Chair Exercises to Promote Relaxation and Reduce Stress in 5 Minutes.

Introduction

Yoga has been a beloved practice for centuries, known for its holistic approach to well-being. In recent years, new discoveries have been introduced to the practice, one of which is the yoga chair. The yoga chair is a versatile and innovative addition to the yoga world, offering support and assistance for practitioners of all levels. This book is dedicated to seniors that require a modified approach to excising in a less stressful on joints. *Senior-Cize : Yoga Chair edition* explores the many benefits of using a yoga chair in your practice, as well as providing guidance and insights on how to use it effectively.

Chapter 1:

UNDERSTANDING THE YOGA CHAIR

In this chapter, we introduce the yoga chair and its purpose in yoga practice. We discuss its design, common features, and materials used to create a stable and supportive chair. You'll learn how the chair is an effective tool for deepening stretches, enhancing alignment, and providing stability during challenging poses.

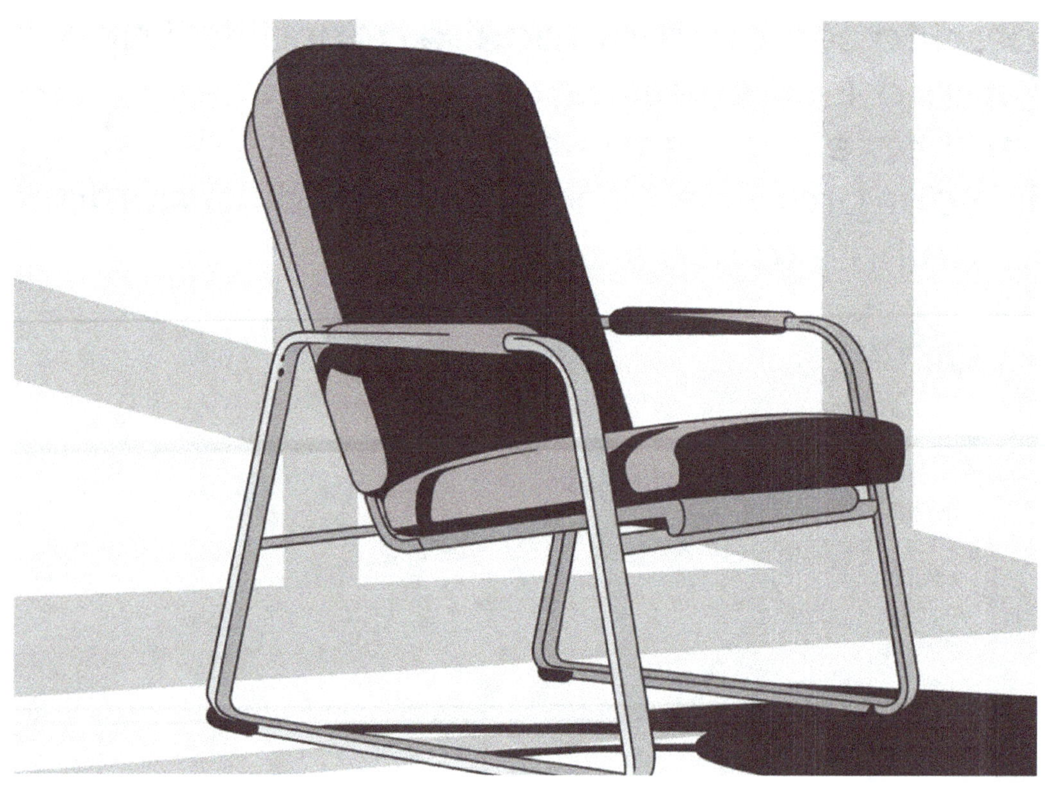

IS CHAIR YOGA GOOD FOR YOU?

For seniors, regular exercise is one of the best ways to achieve a healthy lifestyle. Unlike high-impact exercise like running, lifting weights, and plyometrics, chair yoga is easy on your joints, and may serve as a gateway to other forms of exercise. Chair yoga is a beneficial form of yoga for any fitness level, from active seniors to those recovering from an injury.

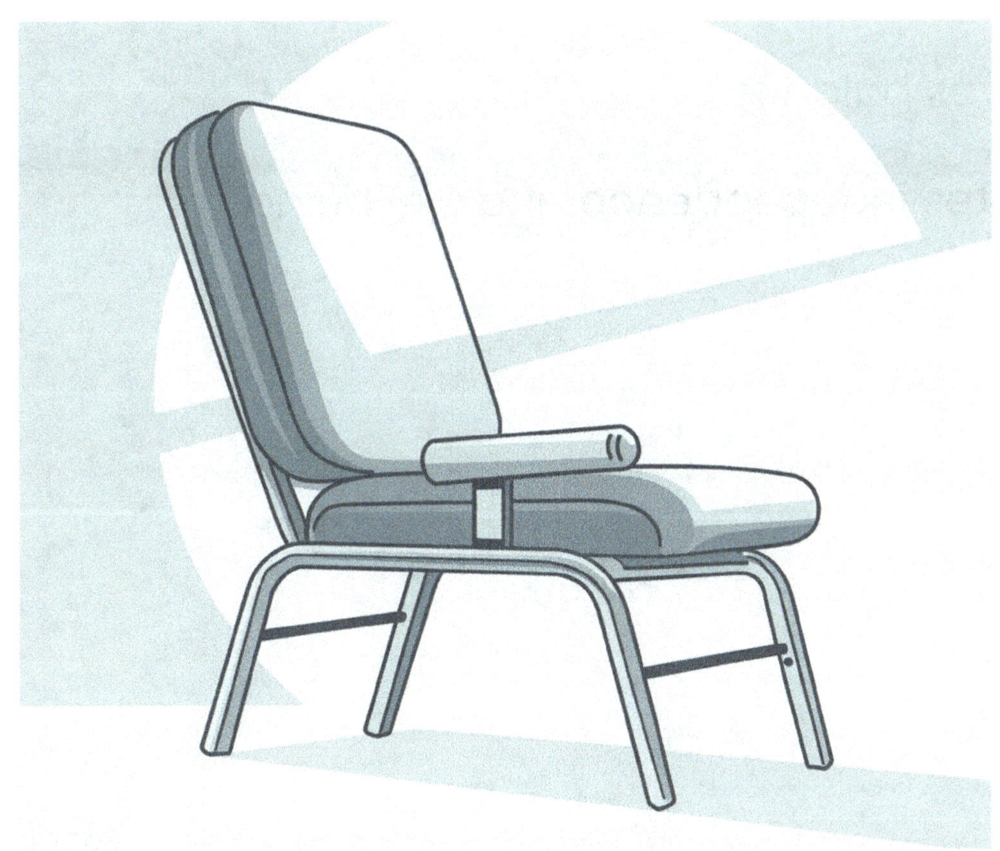

Chair yoga has the following benefits for older adults:

- Low impact on joints

- Improves flexibility

- Stress reduction

- Improves pain management

- Improves circulation

- Combats depression and anxiety

- Improves balance

- Promotes independence and wellbeing

WHAT DOES CHAIR YOGA MEAN?

Chair yoga is a gentle practice in which postures are performed while seated and/or with the aid of a chair. Chair yoga classes typically target those with physical disabilities or aging men and women who find a typical yoga session too challenging. It is also a great form of yoga for beginners or anyone who wants to focus on a gentle practice.

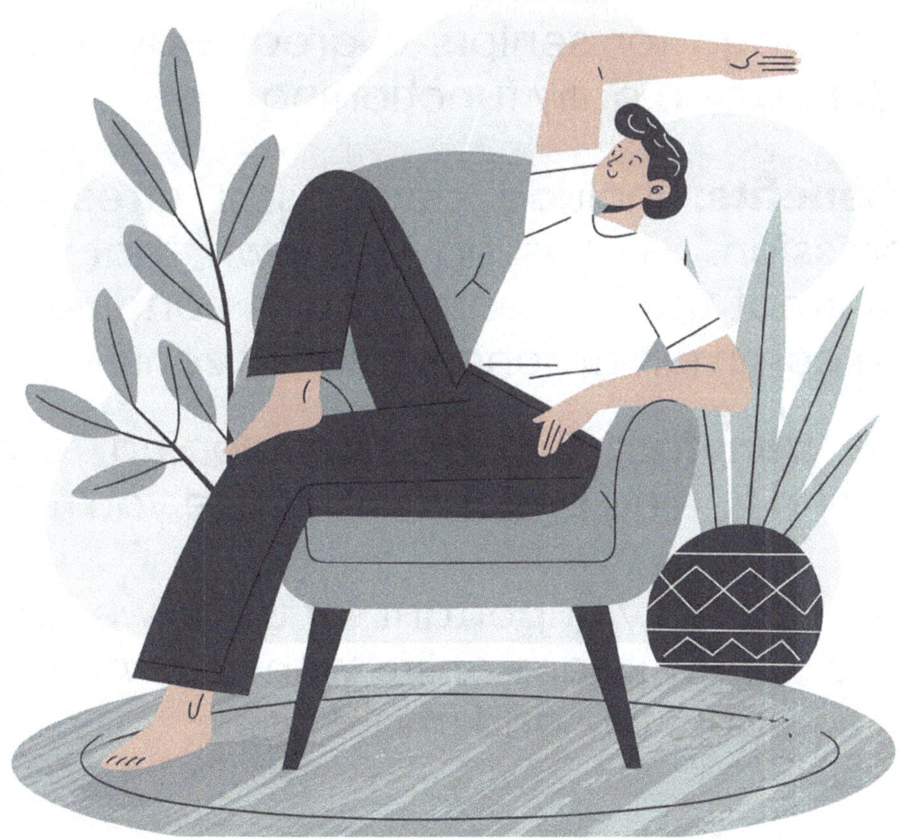

THERE ARE PHYSICAL, MENTAL, AND EMOTIONAL BENEFITS

When you think about exercising, you're usually only expecting to improve your physical health. But with yoga, there are also mental and emotional health benefits.

- **Physical benefits:** include increased strength, flexibility, and balance. Over time, you might also notice you feel less joint pain and are sleeping better. All of these make chair yoga for seniors a great way to maintain independence and daily functioning.

- **Mental benefits:** include decreased stress, anxiety, and depression. Studies have shown that yoga can effectively treat these mental health conditions, which tend to be common among senior citizens.

- **Emotional benefits:** include developing emotional resilience and finding peace with where you're at in life.

These are especially important for us as we age and encounter a new phase of life with its own unique qualities and challenges.

CHAIR YOGA BENEFITS

Chair yoga is a safe and accessible version of traditional yoga for older adults or anyone with mobility challenges.

Chair yoga can:

- **Offer a low-impact workout:** Low-impact exercise is easier on the body. And it's a good exercise option if you have age-related changes in your joints and muscles. You can still get a good workout without injuring yourself or exacerbating old injuries.

- **Boost muscle strength:** Pumping iron isn't the only way to build muscle. This 2016 study shows that yoga is as good as traditional strength training for improving functional fitness. Keep your muscles engaged throughout chair yoga poses. Slowly work your way up to more challenging poses to build strength.

- **Enhance flexibility and joint health:** Yoga is one of the best exercises to keep your muscles flexible and your joints mobile as you age. Maintaining flexibility and mobility helps you stay independent and prevents life-threatening falls.

- **Improve balance:** Poor balance is one of the main reasons for falls in older adults. You can use chair yoga to build a foundation of balance. For example, you can progress by performing the seated yoga poses (as shown below) while standing with the support of a chair. This is one way to slowly improve your balance.

- **Provide a mood boost:** As a mind-body exercise, yoga is well-known for its ability to enhance mood. Yoga offers stress relief, and improves mental and emotional well-being. It also helps with sleep, which is crucial to maintaining a positive mood.

- **Help with chronic conditions:** Yoga may be an effective supplement to regular medical treatment. It can help treat chronic conditions like heart disease, stroke, and chronic obstructive pulmonary disease (COPD), according to a 2015 research review.

- **Relieve aches and pains:** The stretching and strengthening movements of yoga have been shown to improve symptoms of fibromyalgia, low back pain, and neck pain.

COMMON RISKS AND HOW TO NAVIGATE THEM SAFELY

Generally, chair yoga is a low-risk activity. But there are still some potential safety concerns to keep in mind, such as slipping, overstretching, or improper posture. Know common risks and how to practice yoga safely, including:

- Using a chair that is sturdy and does not have wheels to avoid slipping

- Moving gradually and gently to avoid overextension or injury

- Listening to your body so you don't accidentally overstretch or push yourself too hard

- Checking your form to make sure you have proper alignment, which will give you the greatest benefit and help avoid injury

Chapter 2:

BENEFITS OF USING A YOGA CHAIR

Here, we explore the numerous benefits of incorporating a yoga chair into your practice:

• **Enhanced Accessibility:** A yoga chair makes yoga accessible to people with limited mobility, injuries, or disabilities. It provides support and stability, making it easier for practitioners to engage in poses and movements.

• **Improved Flexibility:** The chair can be used to assist with stretching and opening up different areas of the body. It allows practitioners to ease into poses they might not otherwise be able to achieve.

• **Better Posture and Alignment:** By providing support and assistance, the chair can help improve posture and alignment, reducing the risk of injury and promoting proper body mechanics.

• **Increased Strength and Balance:** The chair can be used to target specific muscle groups and challenge balance, enhancing overall strength and stability.

• **Adaptability for All Levels:** The yoga chair can be used by beginners and advanced practitioners alike, offering variations and modifications to suit different skill levels.

Chapter 3:

HOW TO USE A YOGA CHAIR

This chapter provides practical guidance on how to incorporate a yoga chair into your practice. We offer tips on proper setup, safety precautions, and specific poses that can be enhanced with the chair. You'll learn how to use the chair for seated poses, standing poses, and even inversions.

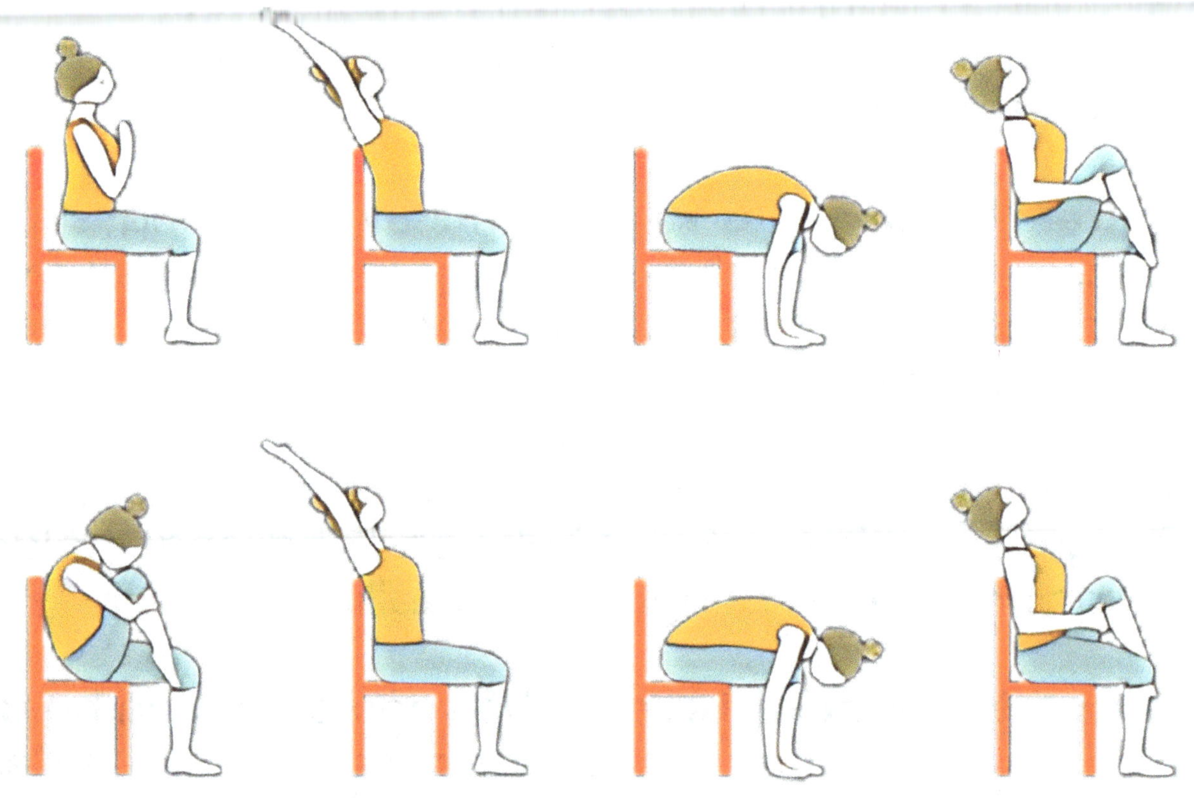

Chapter 4:

YOGA CHAIR SEQUENCES

Here, we present a variety of yoga chair sequences designed for different goals, such as relaxation, strength-building, and flexibility. Each sequence includes detailed instructions and illustrations to guide you through the practice.

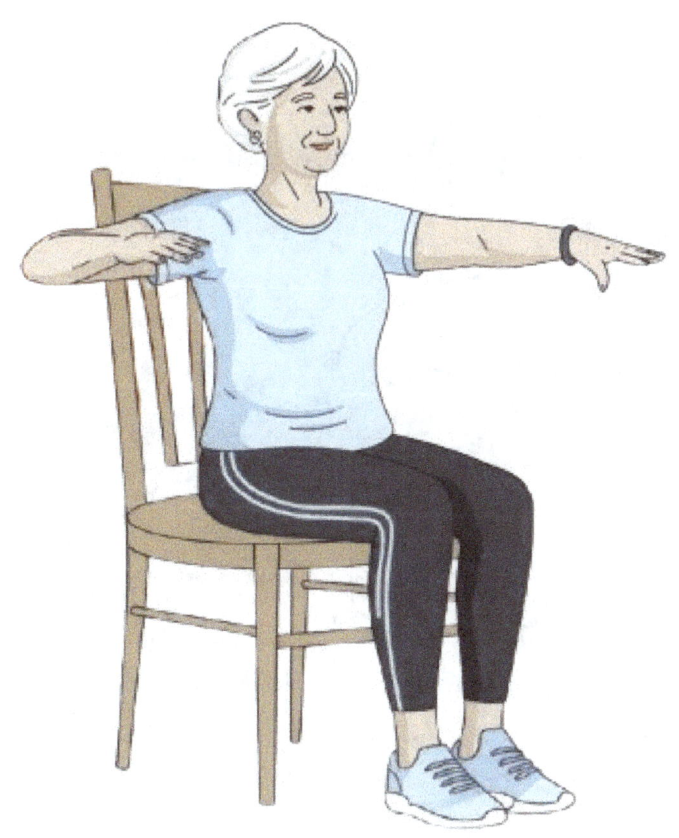

Chapter 5:

SPECIAL CONSIDERATIONS AND MODIFICATIONS

In this chapter, we discuss special considerations for using a yoga chair, such as adapting the practice for pregnancy, injury recovery, and different body types. We also explore ways to modify poses using the chair for individual needs.

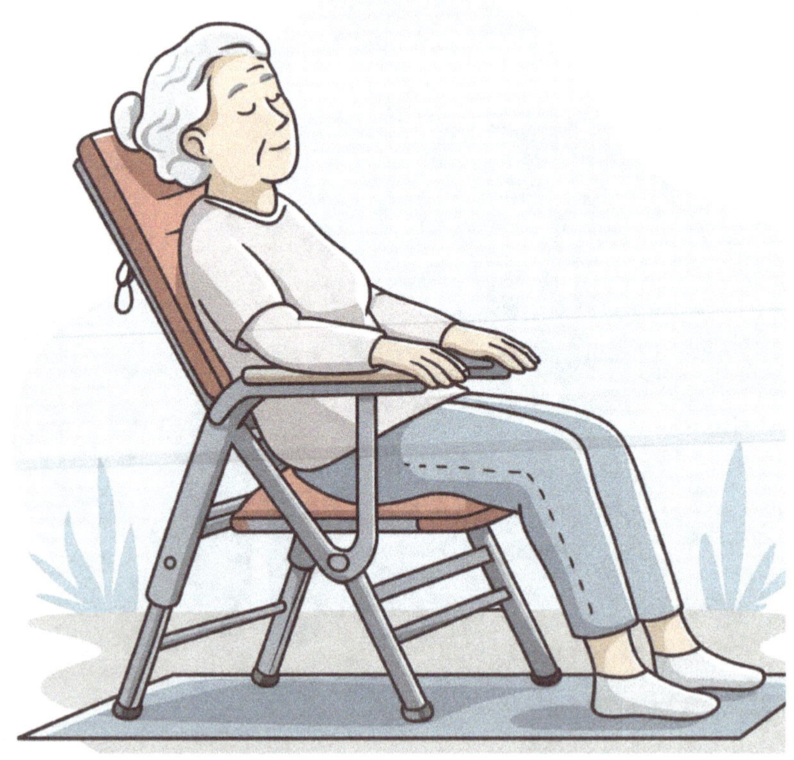

Chapter 6:

CONCLUSION AND RESOURCES

In the final chapter, we summarize the key benefits of using a yoga chair and encourage readers to explore its potential in their practice. We also provide a list of additional resources for further learning and exploration, including recommended books, videos, and websites.

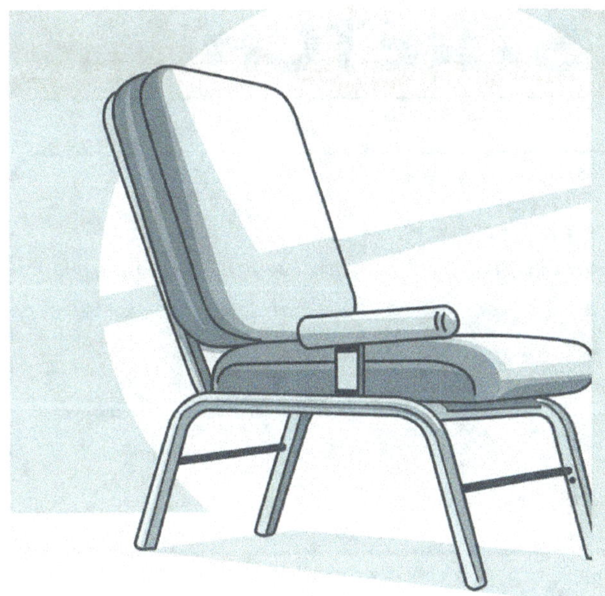

Key benefits

- increased circulation
- feelings of well-being
- decreases in blood pressure

- Decreases anxiety
- Decreases inflammation
- Decreases chronic pain

Appendix

YOGA CHAIR POSES REFERENCE GUIDE

The appendix includes a comprehensive reference guide of yoga chair poses, complete with illustrations and descriptions. This section serves as a quick and easy resource for practitioners to refer to during their practice.

OVERHEAD STRETCH

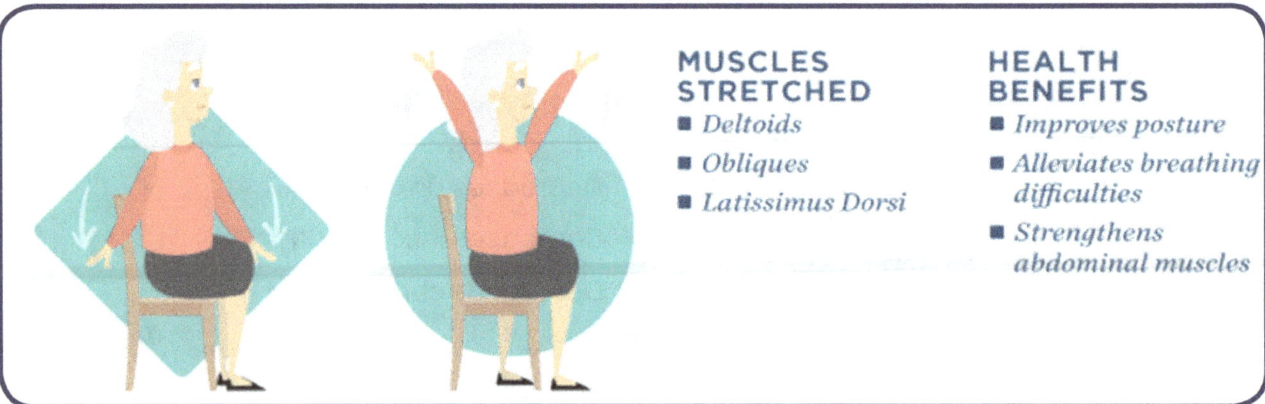

Begin in a cushioned seated position, facing forward with your arms down by your sides. Take a long, deep breath in and slowly stretch your arms upward to the ceiling. Hold this position for a moment, and bring your arms back downward with a long exhale. Throughout this exercise, make sure your core is engaged and your back is as straight as possible.

NECK STRETCH

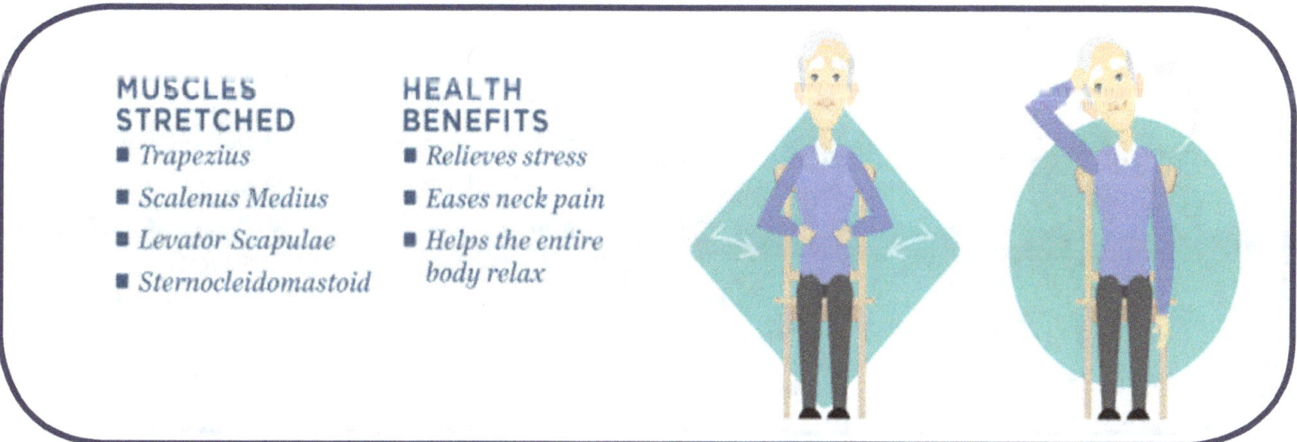

Sit up straight in your chair, and do not let your back touch the back of your chair. Extend your neck slowly upward so you feel the crown of your head rising towards the ceiling. While holding the base of your chair with your right hand, slowly reach upwards with your left hand to hold your left temple.

Take a deep breath, and upon exhalation, gently dip your left ear towards your left shoulder without bending your back or raising your right shoulder. Take several slow breaths in and out in this position, before alternating this stretch to the opposite side.

REVERSE ARM HOLD

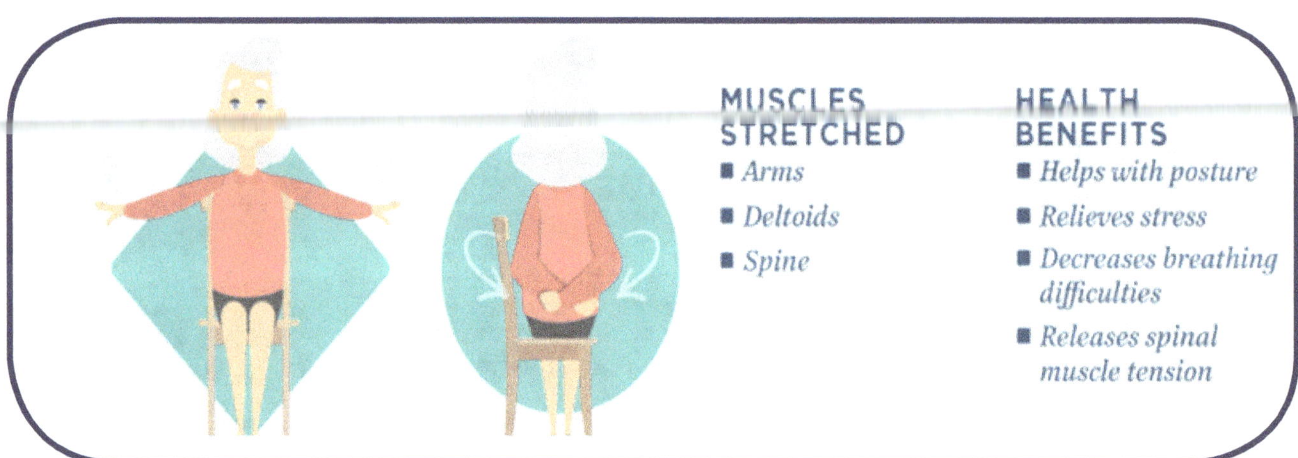

Begin this pose in a seated position with your back straight and apart from the back of the chair. While you inhale deeply, reach your arms straight out to your sides at a low and wide angle. Exhale slowly and reach your hands behind your back, bending your elbows slightly. Arch your back slightly to feel the stretch in your shoulders, and take several breaths in and out.

EAGLE ARMS

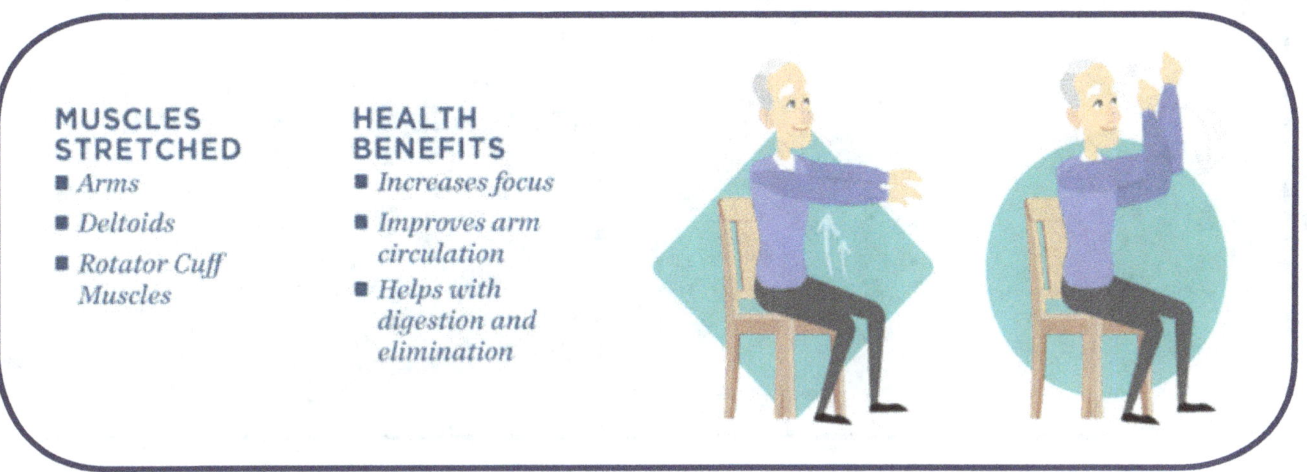

Sit upright in your chair and stretch your arms straight out in front of you. Cross your left arm over your right arm, and bend your elbows to bring your forearms together. Interlace your fingers and raise your elbows slightly, arching your back a bit. Hold this position for several deep breaths. Upon completion, switch to your right arm over your left arm.

CHAIR WARRIOR

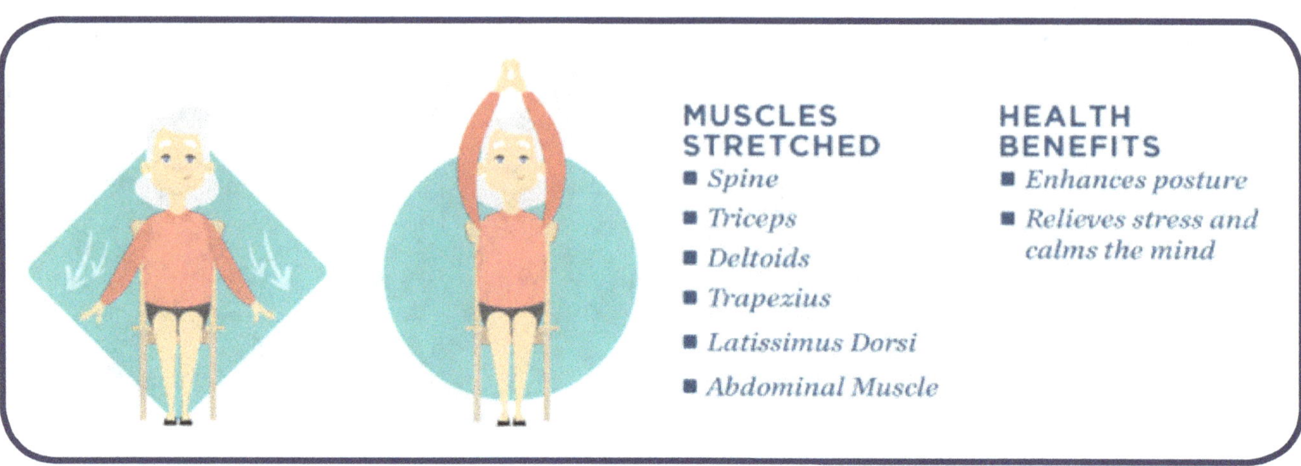

Begin this pose facing forward with your arms down by your side at a wide and low angle, or with one leg across the chair with your torso turned forward (if you're flexible enough for this position). Take a deep breath and slowly raise your arms straight above your head. Hold this pose for several breaths before lowering your arms back down to your sides. If you began this pose with your leg across the chair, switch to the opposite leg across the chair and perform this pose again.

CAT-COW STRETCH

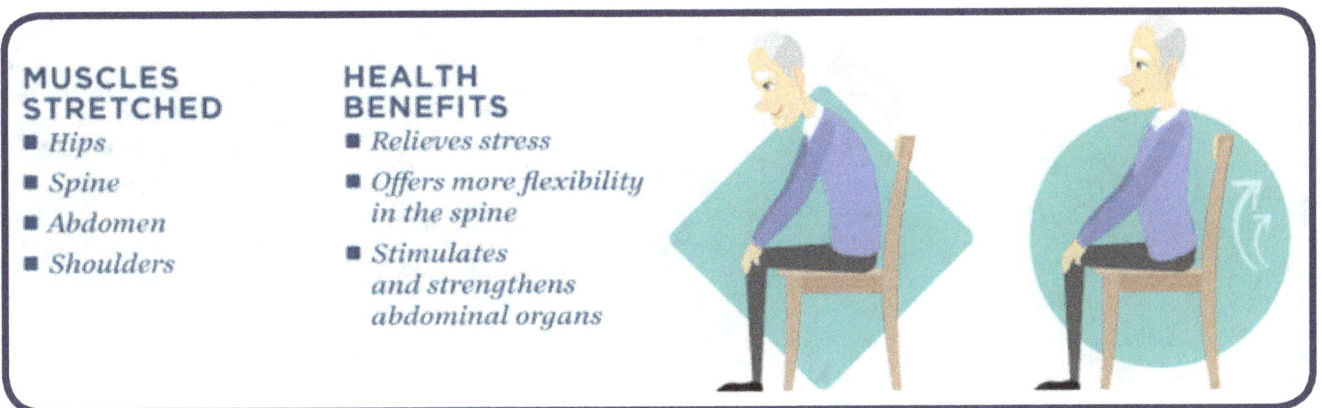

Sit at the edge of your chair with your back as straight as it can be and your core muscles engaged. Inhale and gently arch your back as far as is comfortable for the **"cow"** portion of the stretch, holding the position for three to five breaths.

Then bring your back to its original position, and invert the stretch for the **"cat"** position. Your shoulders will be directly above your hips, but your back will curve into a forward arch. Hold this position for several breaths before returning to your original seated position.

CHAIR SPINAL TWIST

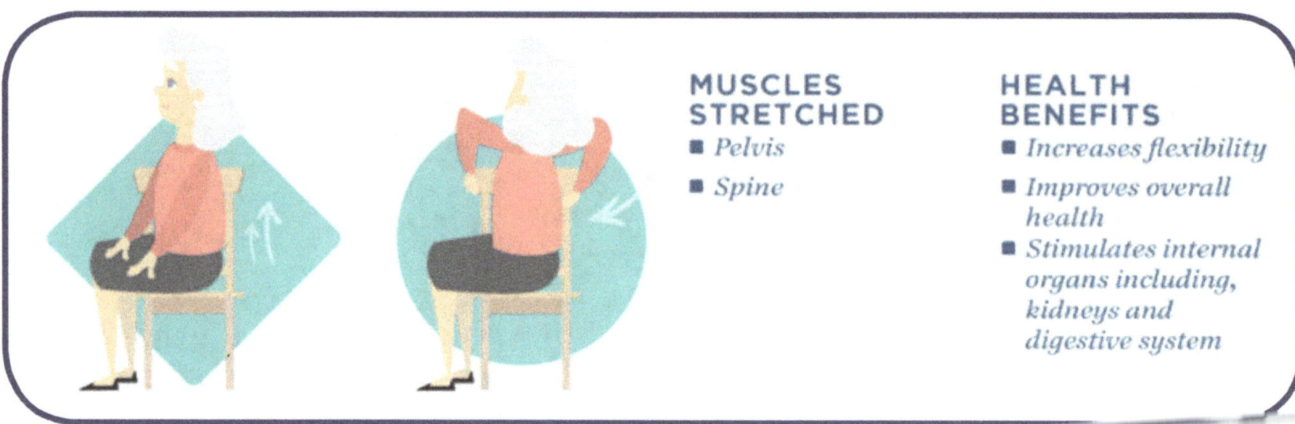

Begin this pose sitting sideways in your chair, with your knees over the right side of the chair and the back of the chair next to your right arm. Make sure your back is straight, and your body is apart from the back of the chair. Hold the back of the chair with both hands, inhale deeply, and slowly turn your body toward the back of the chair while exhaling. Hold this position for several breaths before returning to the original position. After this pose is complete, switch to the other side of the chair, so your knees are over the left side of the chair and the back of the chair is next to your left arm.

SEATED MOUNTAIN

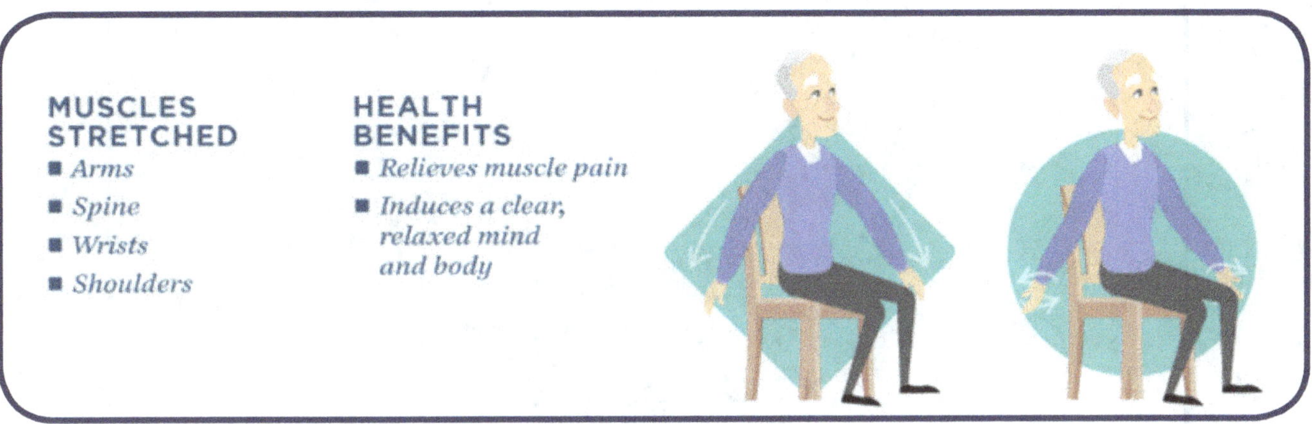

MUSCLES STRETCHED
- *Arms*
- *Spine*
- *Wrists*
- *Shoulders*

HEALTH BENEFITS
- *Relieves muscle pain*
- *Induces a clear, relaxed mind and body*

Start this pose sitting on the front half of your chair with a straight back and an engaged core. Bend your knees at 90-degree angles with your knees above your ankles and a small space between your knees. Inhale slowly and roll your shoulders downward upon exhaling. Activate your abdominal muscles and hold your arms down at your sides. Hold the pose for several deep breaths.

CHAIR CAMEL POSE

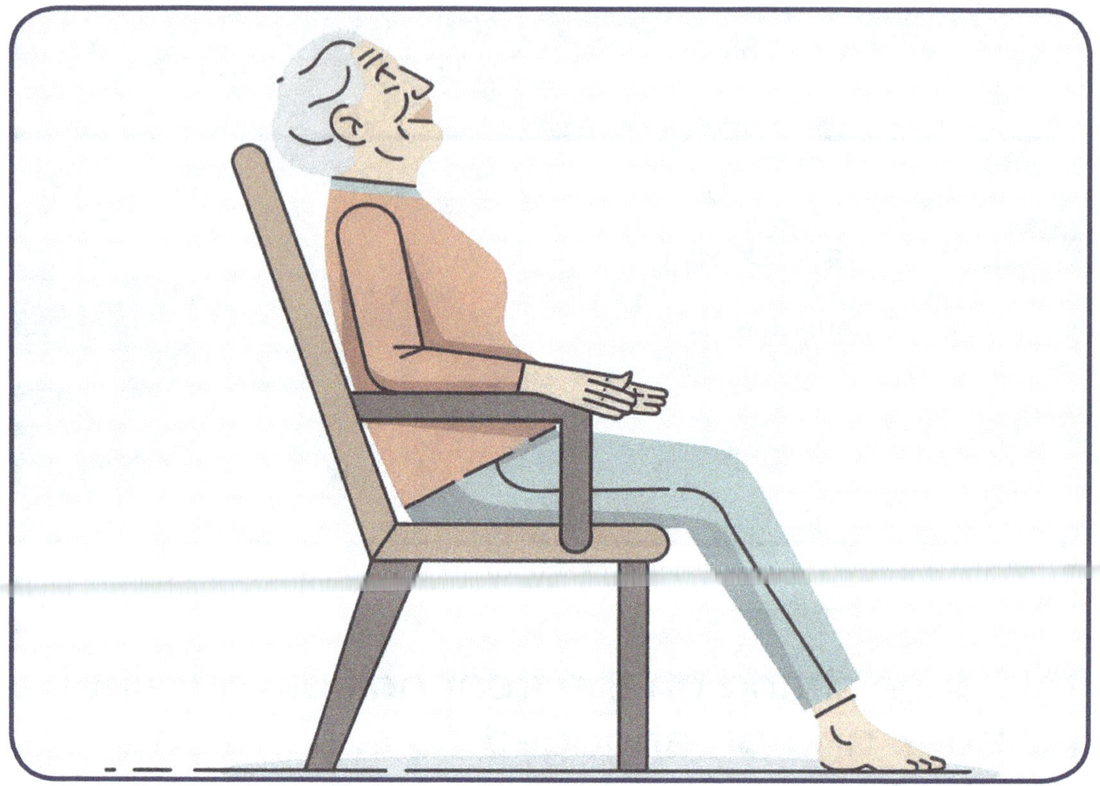

Camel is a backbending posture that stretches the front of your body, including your abdominals and chest. It also strengthens the back muscles.

Step 1: Sit in your chair facing forward.

Step 2: Scoot your hips forward so you are sitting near the edge of your chair. For stability, keep your feet under your knees and not behind them.

Step 3: Inhale, and bring your arms out and around your back, placing your hands in the small of your back. Your fingers should be facing down toward the seat of your chair.

Step 4: Exhale, then inhale again and push your chest out and up to the ceiling. Allow your back to arch, and drop your head back slightly.

Step 5: Keep your neck long and hold this pose while taking several slow, deep breaths. Slowly straighten your spine, and come back to your starting position.

CHAIR FORWARD FOLD

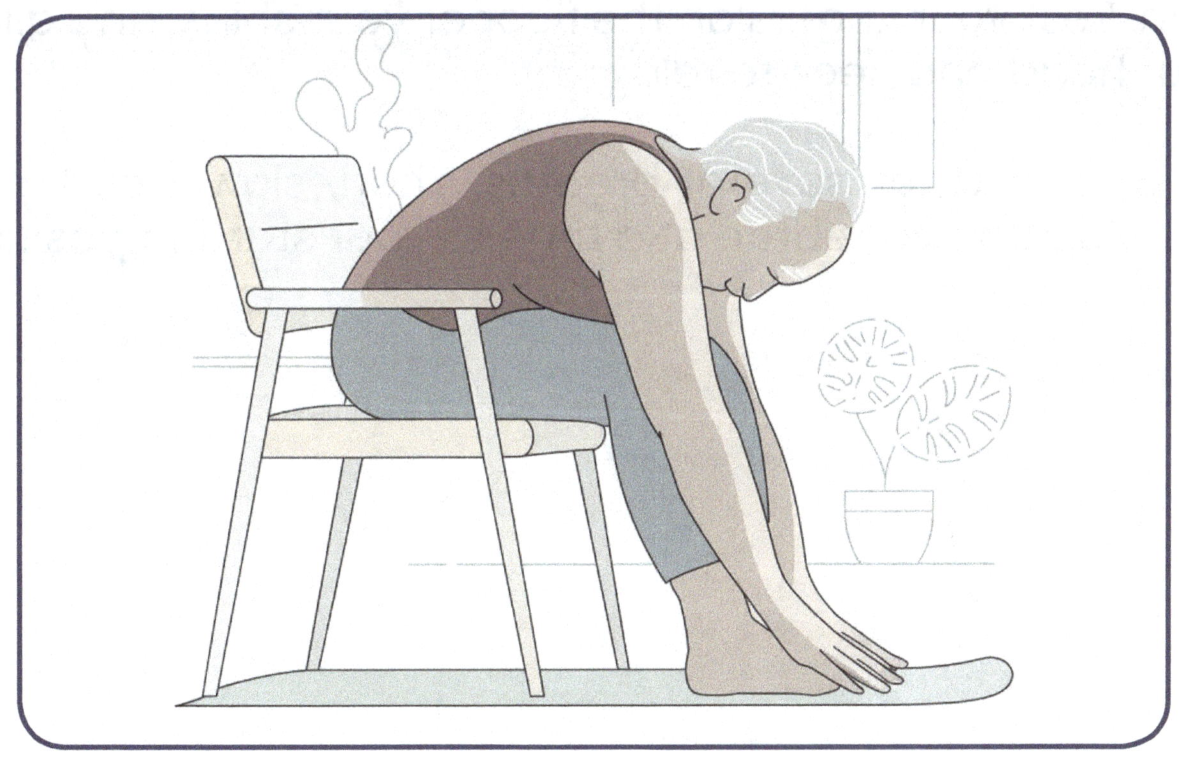

Forward folding poses stretch your entire back body. They are also a type of inversion pose because your head is below your heart. Inversions promote healthy circulation.

Step 1: Sit up tall with your feet flat.

Step 2: Inhale and bring your arms up over your head, parallel to each other.

Step 3: Exhale as you fold forward. As you bend, keep your spine straight and move from your hips rather than rounding your back.

Step 4: Come down as far as you can without any low back pain. Rest your fingers on the floor or your shins, and allow your head and neck to relax.

Step 5: Hold for several breaths. Then, slowly curl your spine up one vertebrae at a time to your starting position.

BREATHING EXERCISES

When practicing senior breathing, particularly during exercise, there are a few things to consider in order to avoid harm and ensure that all of our cells receive oxygen.

Don't hold your breath, to start. Elderly people frequently hold their breath when exercising vigorously.

Second, breathing correctly increases the amount of oxygen we take in.

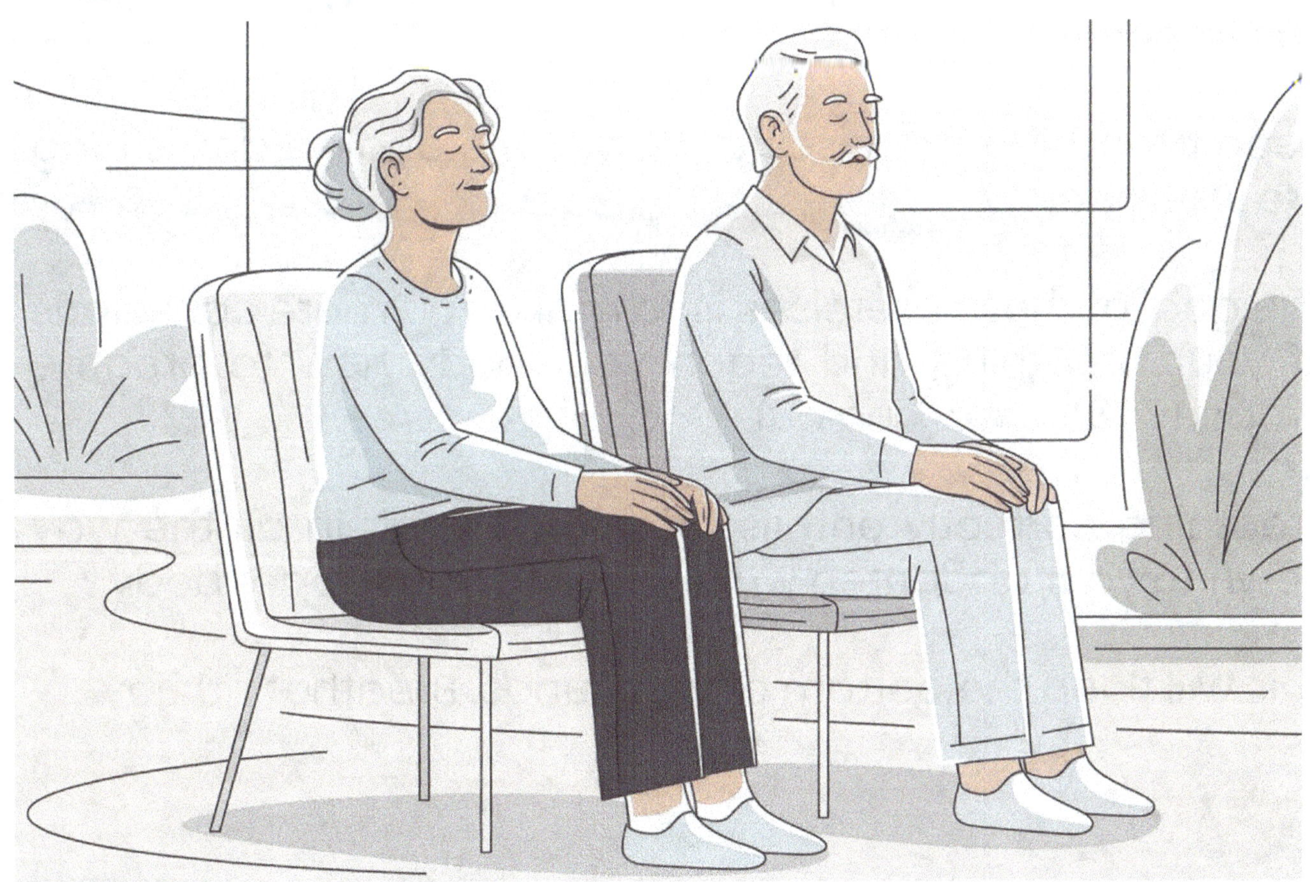

Breathing too shallowly can restrict our capacity to exhale carbon dioxide and absorb oxygen.

It's crucial to have proper posture when standing or sitting when doing deep breathing exercises.

Your lungs can function at their best when you sit with your shoulders back and down, your ribs raised, and your spine in a neutral position.

The lungs need space to expand as air enters. Proper posture increases our pulmonary capacity by allowing the ribs to accept the lungs.

Deep breathing exercises to do while standing and sitting are listed below.

The goal of these exercises is to make you more conscious of your breathing and teach your body how to breathe properly while working out.

Breathing correctly entails bringing the air in all the way down to your abdomen while relaxing your upper body.

This will flood the bottom of your lungs. Breathe with joy.

STEP 1: BREATHING EXERCISE WHILE SITTING

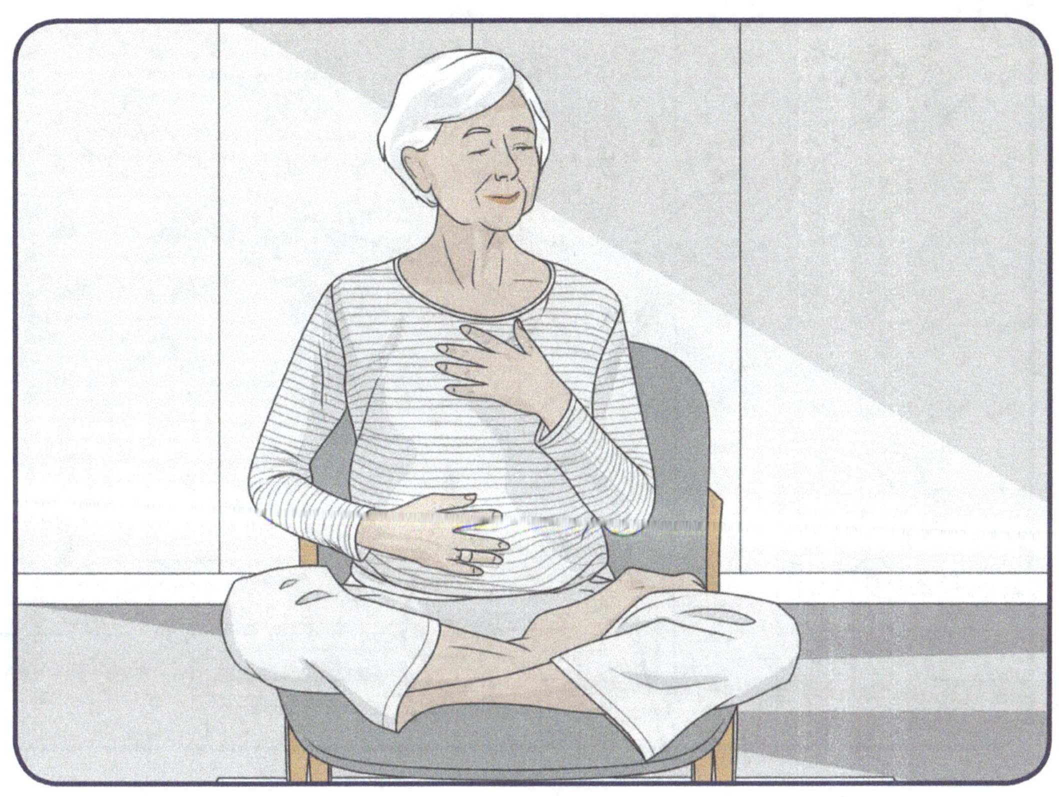

Take a seat comfortably. Put your left hand on your stomach and your right on your chest. Breathe in till your right hand comes up. This type of chest breathing makes utilization of the lungs' upper lobes. Then take a breath that causes your left hand to raise.The lower lobes of the lung are used in this type of abdominal breathing.To get the most out of activity, this is the recommended breathing technique.

STEP 2: BREATHING EXERCISE WHILE STANDING

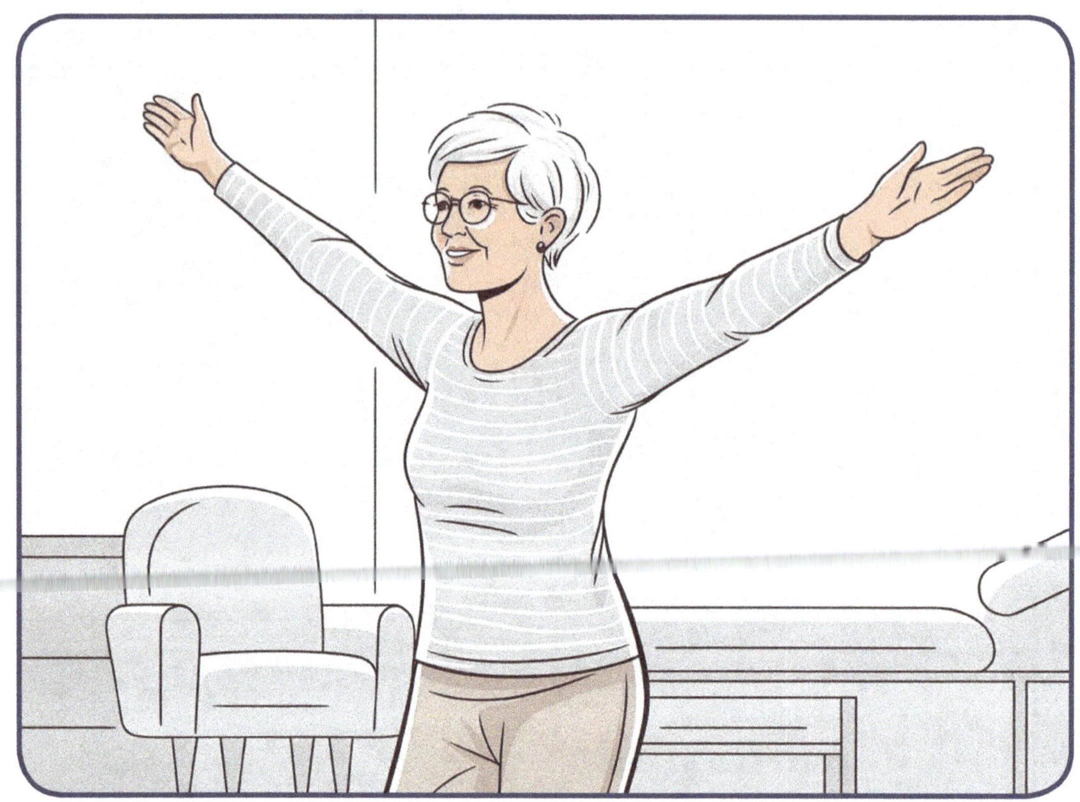

- Place both hands on your belly and stand.

- Inhale deeply, then expand your abdomen.

- This is deep breathing in the lower lobes.

STEP 3: EXERCISE FOR LIFTING THE RIBS

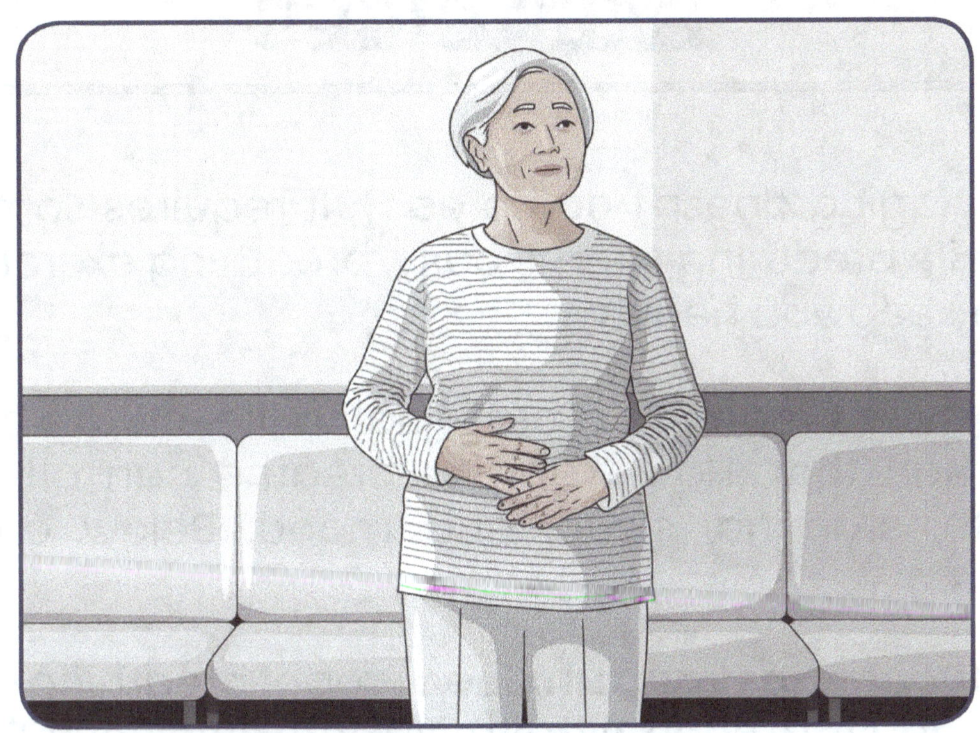

Cross your arms at the wrists in front of your waist as you stand. Lift your arms above your head and take a deep breath. Breathe out and relax while lowering your arms. Do this ten times.

Guidelines

1. Be sure to uphold proper posture while sitting and standing.
2. Maintain your spine in a relaxed neutral alignment.
3. Elevate your ribs and retract your shoulders during your workouts.

BENEFITS OF BREATHING EXERCISES

Healthy aging doesn't come easy. It requires some work. And while breathing seems easy, breathing exercises can help to keep you healthy.

We all know breathing is essential to life, but it's so much more than that. How well you breathe can affect your strength, stamina, sleep, and mood. Below are more benefits.

- **It reduces stress and anxiety:** Proper breathing can help older adults to cope with stress more efficiently. Exercises like deep breathing activate the body's relaxation response, leading to reduced stress hormones and a sense of calm.

- **It may increase lung capacity:** As we age, our lung capacity may decrease. Breathing exercises can help maintain or improve lung function by promoting better oxygen exchange and increasing the efficiency of the respiratory muscles.

- **It improves digestion:** Deep breathing exercises can stimulate the parasympathetic nervous system, which promotes relaxation and aids in digestion. It is especially beneficial if you experience digestive issues.

- **It improves sleep and mood:** Practicing healthy breathing before bed can help you relax your body and mind, leading to more quality sleep. It can also trigger endorphins and other feel-good chemicals in the brain, leading to improved mood and a reduced risk of depression. It calms your mind.

- **It improves your posture:** Practicing breathing can also help you maintain musculoskeletal health and prevent discomfort or pain.

- **Better Oxygenation:** Breathing exercises enhance oxygen intake and distribution throughout your body. This increased oxygenation can improve energy levels, cognitive function, and overall vitality.

The benefits of breathing exercises are numerous, and according to the National Institutes of Health, controlled breathing can be especially beneficial for older adults.

Older adults who don't take the time to breathe deeply can experience ribcage stiffness and muscle weakness, which leads to shallow breaths and a poor oxygen supply.

Shallow breathing can make you feel sluggish and uncomfortable and may even prevent you from maintaining an active lifestyle.

However, just like many functions of your body, lung strength can be significantly improved with regular exercise.

BREATHING EXERCISE'S GOAL

- Boost the health of your lungs.

- Aids in removing pollutants and poisons from the lungs.

- Improves the amount of oxygen in your lungs, which gives you more energy.

WHAT IS MEDITATION?

Simply put, meditation is a practice that involves training the mind to be more present and focused. It typically involves sitting quietly and paying attention to your breath, body, or a particular sound or image to make distractions melt away & bring you wholly into the present moment. If you're picturing yourself trying to twist yourself into a Buddha-like pose—don't worry! You can meditate sitting in a chair, laying down or in any number of postures & positions.

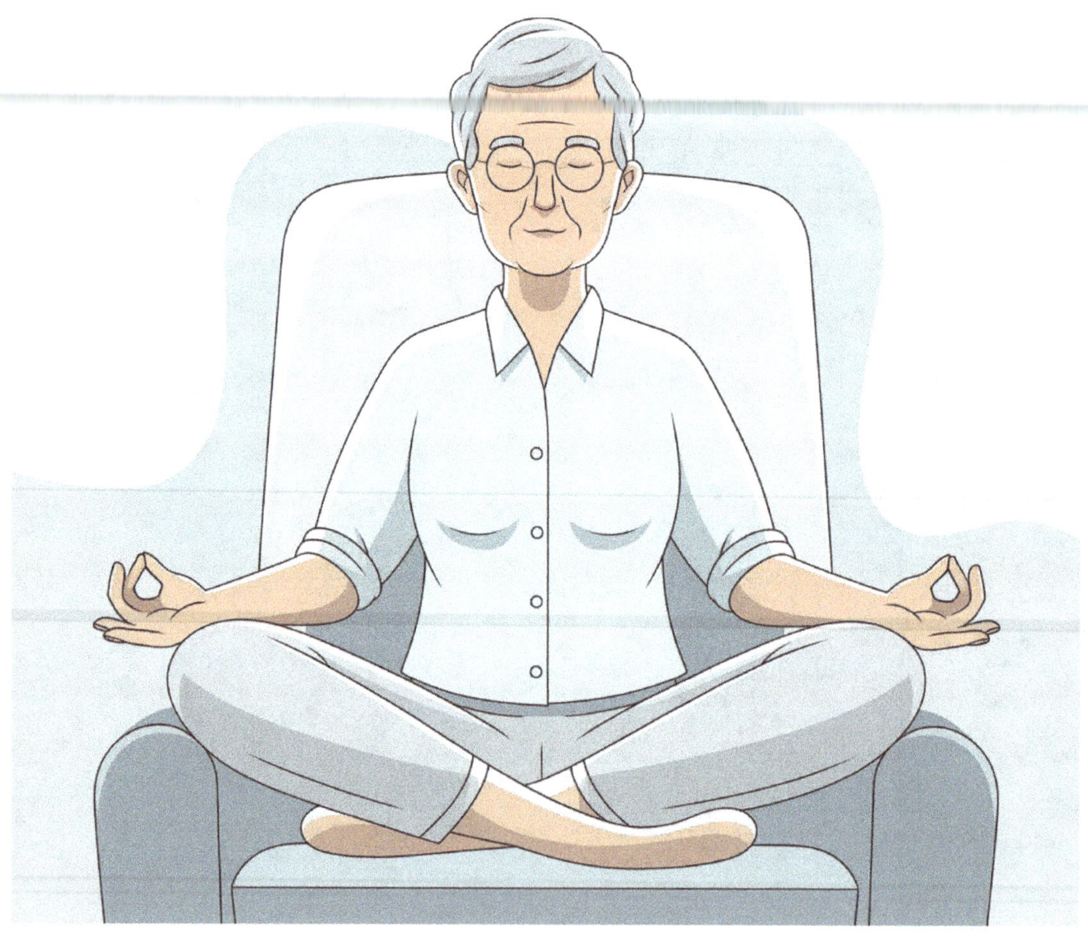

WHY SHOULD SENIORS MEDITATE?

In today's fast-paced world, it's easy to get caught up in a cycle of constant stimulation and distraction. Spending time being present and focused helps us to slow down and reconnect with ourselves. By doing so, you can learn to cultivate a sense of calm and clarity, and develop a greater awareness of your thoughts and emotions.

This can be a powerful tool for reducing stress and anxiety, improving sleep quality, and enhancing overall well-being. It can also help us to become more resilient in the face of challenges, and develop a greater sense of compassion and empathy for ourselves and others.

BEST MEDITATION TECHNIQUES FOR SENIORS

1. Mindfulness Meditation

2. Guided Meditation

3. Body Scan Meditation

4. Gentle Yoga

1. MINDFULNESS MEDITATION

Mindfulness meditation involves focusing on the present moment and paying attention to one's thoughts and emotions without judgment. To practice mindfulness meditation:

- Find a quiet and comfortable space to sit or lie down
- Set a timer for a desired length of time
- Focus on your breath or a specific sensation in your body
- If your mind wanders, gently bring it back to your breath or sensation

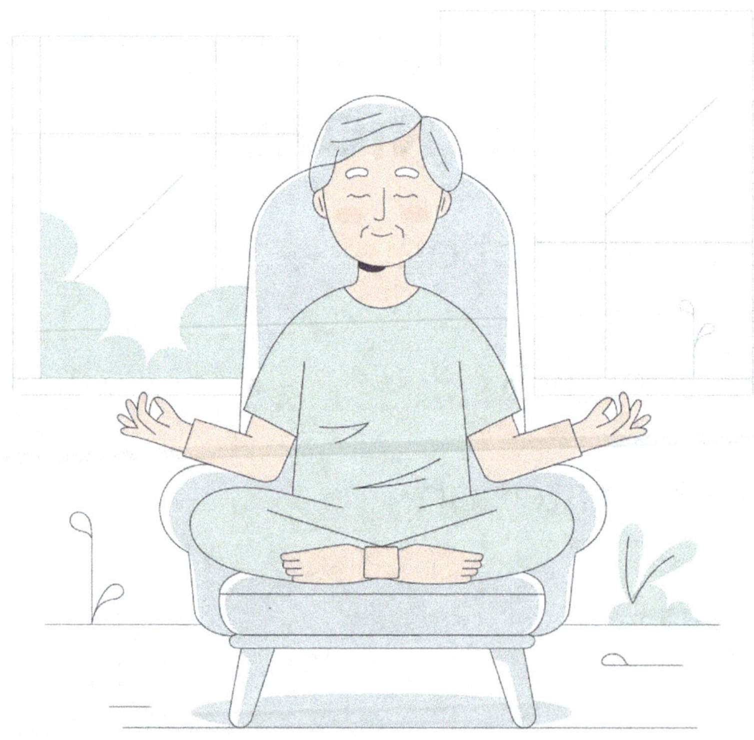

2. GUIDED MEDITATION

Guided meditation involves listening to a meditation guide or teacher who leads the individual through a series of relaxation techniques & visualizations. To practice guided meditation:

- Find a quiet and comfortable space to sit or lie down
- Find a guided meditation resource such as an app or podcast
- Follow along with the guide's instructions

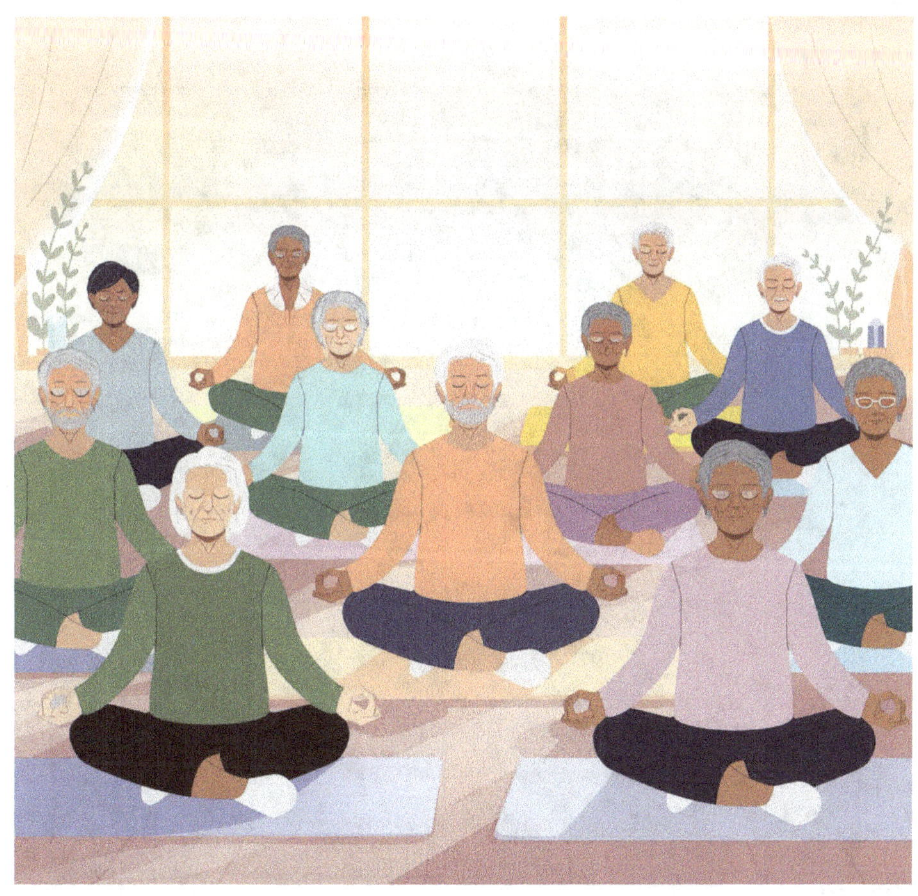

3. BODY SCAN MEDITATION

Body scan meditation involves scanning the body from head to toe and paying attention to any sensations or areas of tension. To practice body scan meditation:

- Find a quiet and comfortable space to lie down
- Start at the top of your head and work your way down your body
- Pay attention to any sensations or areas of tension in each body part
- If you notice tension, try to relax that area by breathing into it

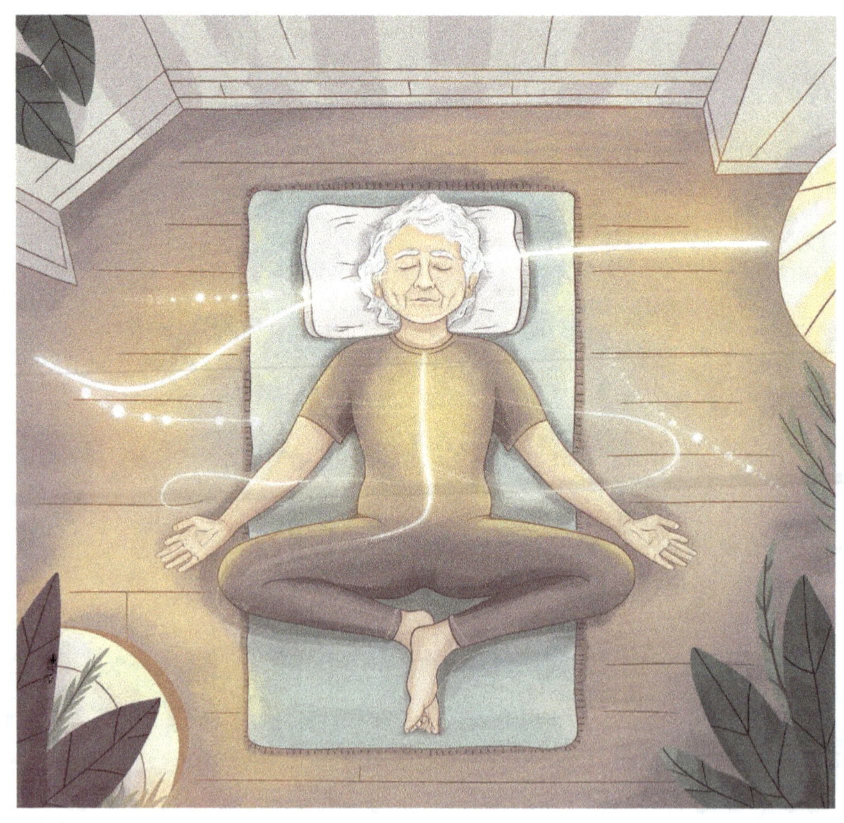

4. GENTLE YOGA

These mindfulness activities involve movement and breath work to increase awareness and reduce stress. To practice gentle yoga, tai chi, or walking meditation:

- Find a quiet and comfortable space to practice
- Follow along with a teacher or video resource
- Focus on your breath and movement

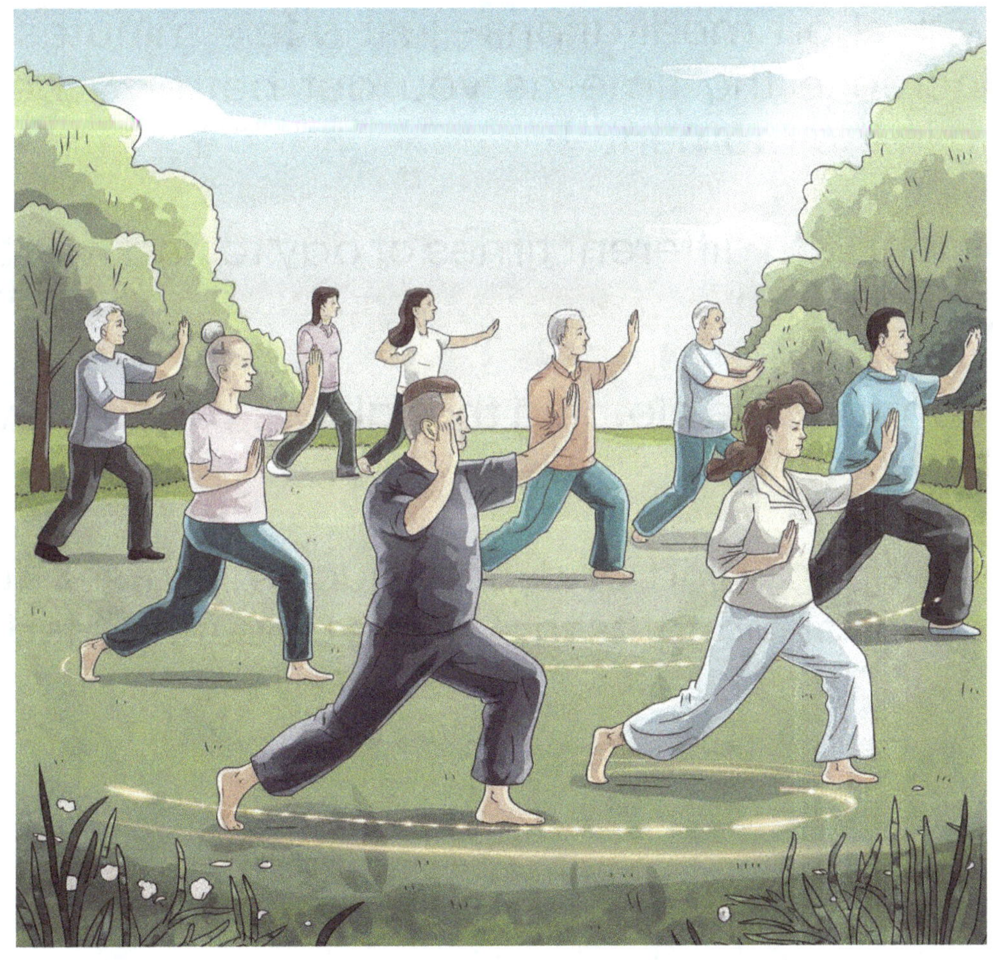

MEDITATION TIPS FOR SENIORS

- Choose a quiet and comfortable space to meditate

- Use props such as cushions, blankets, or chairs for support and comfort—you don't have to break a leg trying to twist your feet into a lotus pose. Choose a position that is truly comfortable for you!

- Start with short meditations—just a few minutes a day, then increase the time as you get better & better at staying in the moment

- Experiment with different times of day to find what works best for you

- Wear comfortable clothing that allows you to move and breathe freely

- Keep an open mind and don't judge yourself for any distractions or thoughts that come up during meditation

MINDFULNESS ACTIVITIES FOR SENIORS

- Engage in mindful breathing exercises

- Try journaling or reflective writing

- Practice gratitude by writing down things you are thankful for

- Spend time in nature and focus on senses

- Try a sensory meditation, such as smelling different scents or tasting different foods

- Engage in art or craft activities mindfully, such as painting, knitting or pottery-making

MEDITATION BENEFITS FOR SENIORS

Meditation helps keep your mind relaxed and engaged, which enables you to age with grace. Meditation can offer some surprising health benefits to seniors who are looking for new pathways to health.

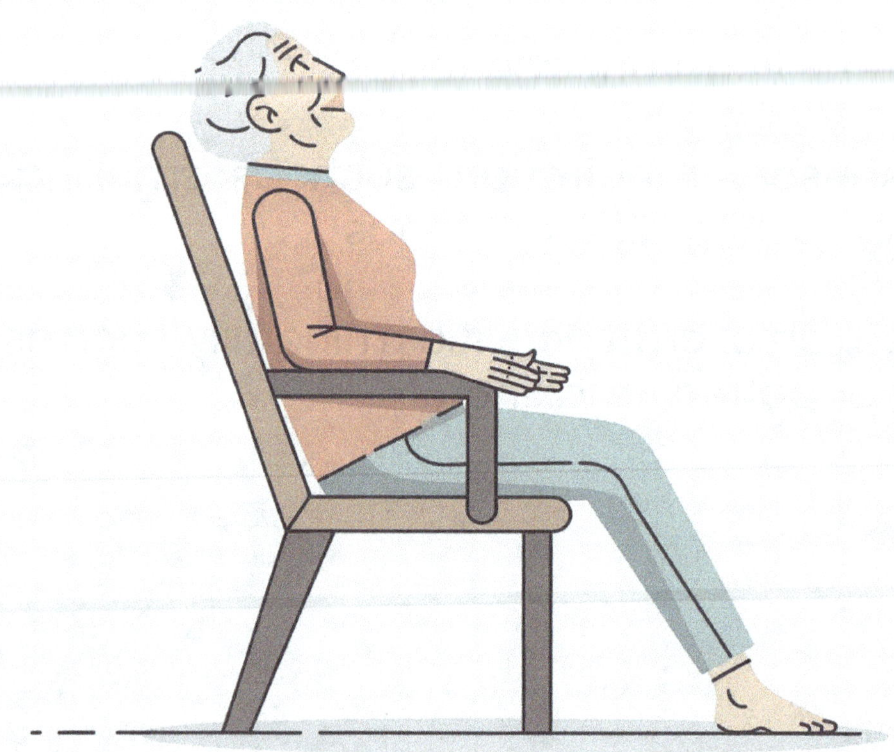

Here are 10 benefits seniors get from meditation:

1. Boosts Immune System
2. Controls Pain
3. Enhances Strength, Flexibility and Balance
4. Helps Stave Off Depression
5. Improves Sleep
6. Increases Attention Span
7. Controls Blood Pressure
8. Promotes Mindfulness
9. Reduces Stress and Anxiety
10. Stabilizes Memory

1. BOOSTS IMMUNE SYSTEM

Meditation appears to suppress damaging processes in the body while boosting cortisol levels, which helps the function of the immune system. This can help treat various inflammatory conditions, such as ulcerative colitis and irritable bowel syndrome.

2. CONTROLS PAIN

Chronic pain increases with age and is highest among seniors 65 and over.

Since our physical perception of pain is directly linked to our minds, it can be raised when we're under a lot of stress. Mindfulness meditation is a great way to control pain because it allows you to focus on breathing and how the body feels in the present moment.

3. ENHANCES STRENGTH, FLEXIBILITY AND BALANCE

Slow, measured movements in meditation and especially yoga poses can lead to better balance and movement, which can also help prevent falls.

Falls are the leading cause of injury among seniors, but yoga can help seniors work on balance and strength to avoid them.

4. HELPS STAVE OFF DEPRESSION

Meditation can boost the mood and help people overcome depression, according to a study published in the Journal of the American Medical Association.

Other research indicates that meditation may be as good as antidepressants to relieve depression in some patients.

5. IMPROVES SLEEP

Sleep problems often stem from stress, poor diet, aging or chronic illnesses. But meditation before bedtime releases tension from your body, creating a peaceful state of mind.

Research published by JAMA Internal Medicine showed that a group who practiced meditation reported less insomnia, fatigue and other such symptoms.

6. INCREASES ATTENTION SPAN

Focused meditation practices can have a tangible effect on the strength and endurance of your attention span. A study published in Frontiers in Human Neuroscience says meditation improves attention even in those who have just started meditation programs.

Over an extended period of time, the study says, there will be positive effects on body awareness, emotion regulation and attention span.

7. CONTROLS BLOOD PRESSURE

Meditation may help those with high blood pressure, according to studies cited by the National Institutes of Health.

These benefits were seen mostly in those with mild hypertension.

8. PROMOTES MINDFULNESS

Seniors can face many stresses as they age, from moving to nursing homes to adjusting to new daily habits. These changes can create stress, so they can benefit from the meditative effects of mindfulness.

Mindfulness meditation for seniors can include yoga or other techniques that teach participants to explore their thoughts and emotions. Practitioners say meditation can help seniors stay connected to the world.

9. REDUCES STRESS AND ANXIETY

During meditation, your mind may be focused on eliminating inner thoughts that tend to cause a strain on your emotional well-being. Having a good state of self-awareness and tranquility will help you manage any symptoms related to stress throughout the day.

10. STABILIZES MEMORY

Meditation can help slow memory loss. According to a study referenced in the Harvard Gazette, mindfulness meditation for at least 30 minutes a day can increase gray matter in the hippocampus. This part of the brain plays an important role in memory and learning.

Other researchers found that people who meditate regularly can harness the power or feeling of a subconscious mind, giving your brain the ability to retain more information.

RELAXATION TECHNIQUES FOR STRESS RELIEF

To effectively combat stress, you need to activate your body's natural relaxation response. Techniques such as deep breathing, visualization, meditation, and yoga can help.

- Deep breathing

- Visuallization

- Self massage

- Rythmic movement and mindful excercise

With its focus on full, cleansing breaths, deep breathing is a simple yet powerful relaxation technique. It's easy to learn, can be practiced almost anywhere, and provides a quick way to get your stress levels in check. Deep breathing is the cornerstone of many other relaxation practices, too, and can be combined with other relaxing elements such as aromatherapy and music. While apps and audio downloads can guide you through the process, all you really need is a few minutes and a place to sit quietly or stretch out.

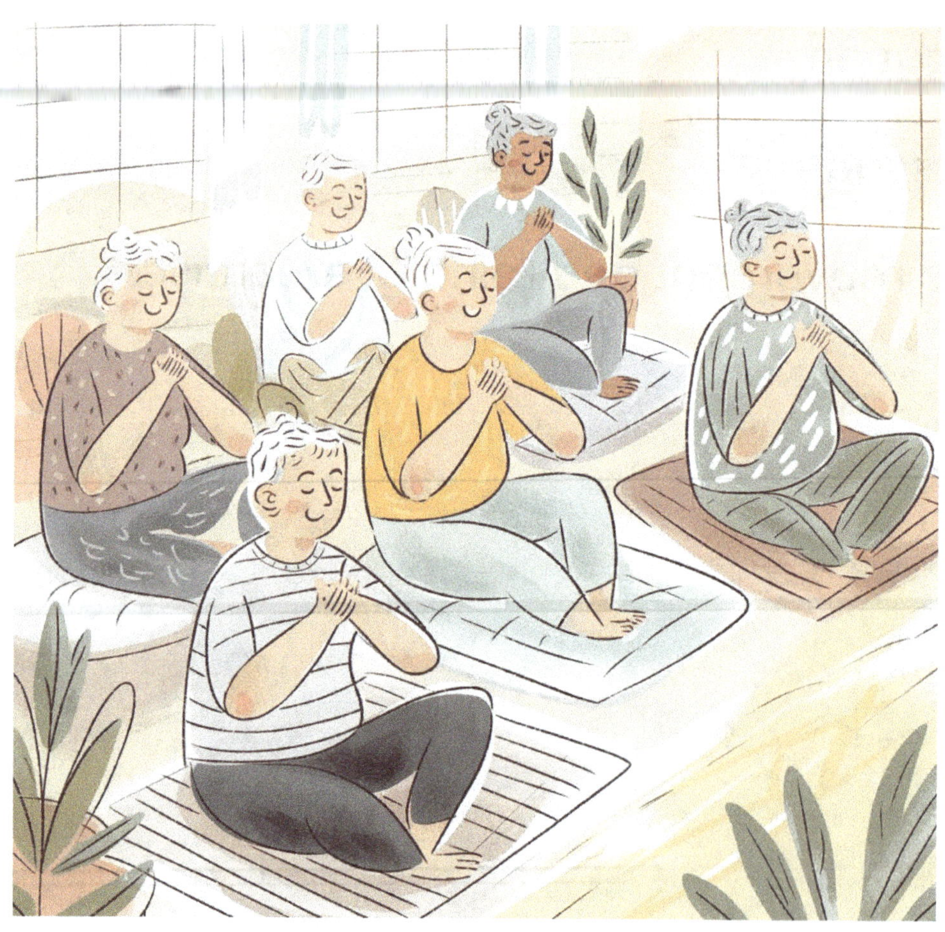

HOW TO PRACTICE DEEP BREATHING

- Sit comfortably with your back straight. Put one hand on your chest and the other on your stomach.

- Breathe in through your nose. The hand on your stomach should rise. The hand on your chest should move very little.

- Exhale through your mouth, pushing out as much air as you can while contracting your abdominal muscles. The hand on your stomach should move in as you exhale, but your other hand should move very little.

- Continue to breathe in through your nose and out through your mouth. Try to inhale enough so that your lower abdomen rises and falls. Count slowly as you exhale.

- If you find it difficult breathing from your abdomen while sitting up, try lying down. Put a small book on your stomach, and breathe so that the book rises as you inhale and falls as you exhale.

2: VISUALIZATION

Visualization, or guided imagery, is a variation on traditional meditation that involves imagining a scene in which you feel at peace, free to let go of all tension and anxiety. Choose whatever setting is most calming to you, whether it's a tropical beach, a favorite childhood spot, or a quiet wooded glen.

You can practice visualization on your own or with an app or audio download to guide you through the imagery. You can also choose to do your visualization in silence or use listening aids, such as soothing music or a sound machine or a recording that matches your chosen setting: the sound of ocean waves if you've chosen a beach, for example.

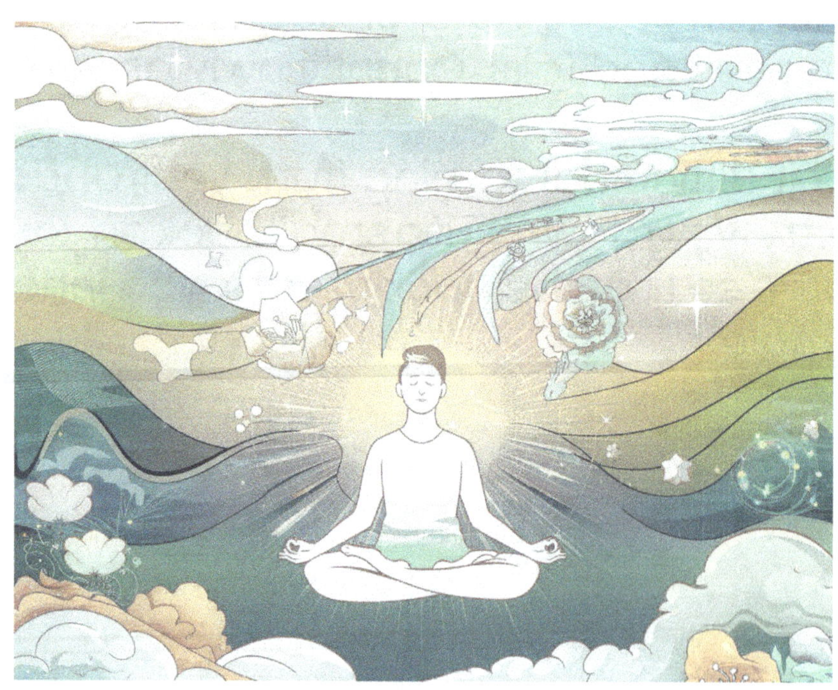

PRACTICING VISUALIZATION

Close your eyes and imagine your restful place. Picture it as vividly as you can: everything you see, hear, smell, taste, and feel. Just "looking" at it in your mind's eye like you would a photograph is not enough. Visualization works best if you incorporate as many sensory details as possible. For example, if you are thinking about a dock on a quiet lake:

- See the sun setting over the water
- Hear the birds singing
- Smell the pine trees
- Feel the cool water on your bare feet
- Taste the fresh, clean air

Enjoy the feeling of your worries drifting away as you slowly explore your restful place. When you are ready, gently open your eyes and come back to the present. Don't worry if you sometimes zone out or lose track of where you are during a visualization session. This is normal. You may also experience feelings of heaviness in your limbs, muscle twitches, or yawning. Again, these are normal responses.

3: SELF-MASSAGE

You're probably already aware how much a professional massage at a spa or health club can help reduce stress, relieve pain, and ease muscle tension. What you may not be aware of is that you can experience some of the same benefits at home or work by practicing self-massage, trading massages with a loved one, or using an adjustable bed with a built-in massage feature.

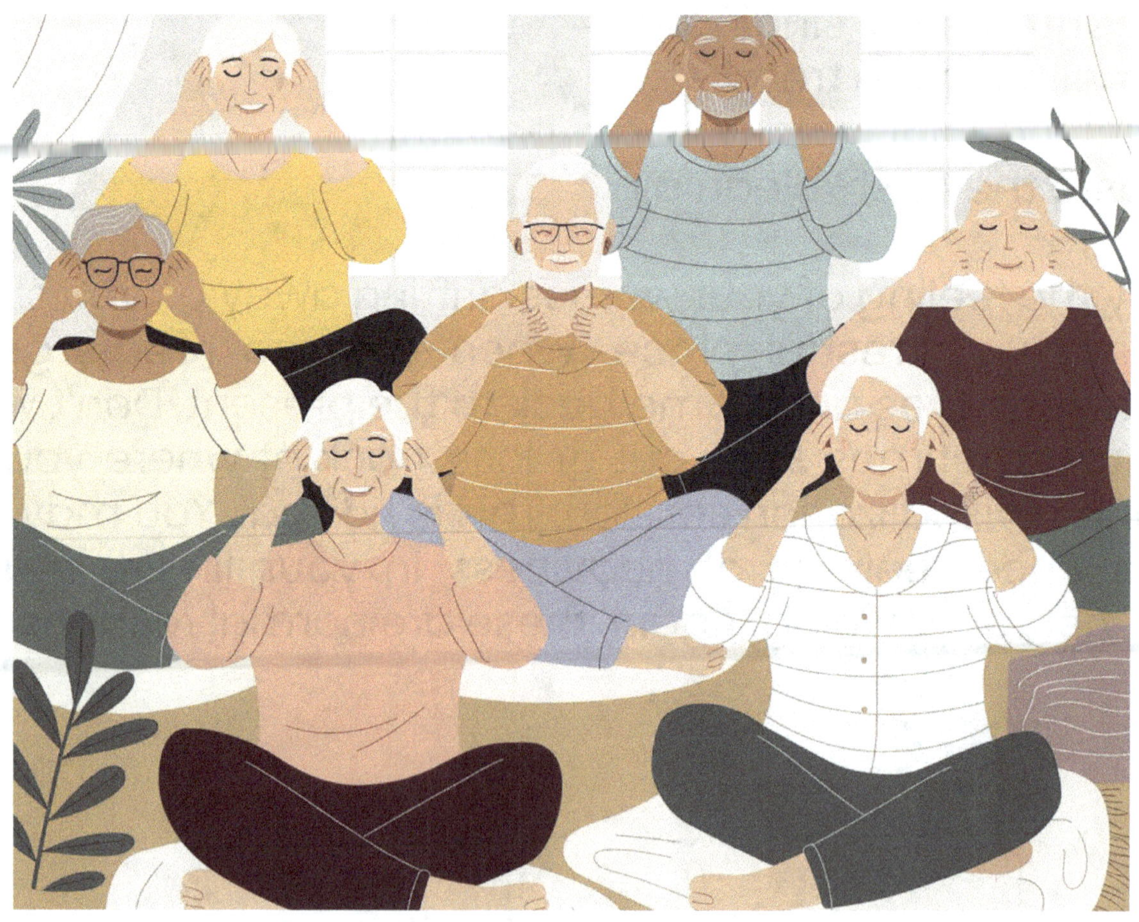

A FIVE-MINUTE SELF-MASSAGE TO RELIEVE STRESS

A combination of strokes works well to relieve muscle tension. Try gentle chops with the edge of your hands or tapping with fingers or cupped palms. Put fingertip pressure on muscle knots. Knead across muscles, and try long, light, gliding strokes. You can apply these strokes to any part of the body that falls easily within your reach. For a short session like this, try focusing on your neck and head:

- Start by kneading the muscles at the back of your neck and shoulders. Make a loose fist and drum swiftly up and down the sides and back of your neck. Next, use your thumbs to work tiny circles around the base of your skull. Slowly massage the rest of your scalp with your fingertips. Then tap your fingers against your scalp, moving from the front to the back and then over the sides.

- Now massage your face. Make a series of tiny circles with your thumbs or fingertips. Pay particular attention to your temples, forehead, and jaw muscles. Use your middle fingers to massage the bridge of your nose and work outward over your eyebrows to your temples.

- Finally, close your eyes. Cup your hands loosely over your face and inhale and exhale easily for a short while.

4: RHYTHMIC MOVEMENT AND MINDFUL EXERCISE

The idea of exercising may not sound particularly soothing, but rhythmic exercise that gets you into a flow of repetitive movement can produce the relaxation response. Examples include:

- Running
- Walking
- Swimming
- Dancing
- Rowing
- Climbing

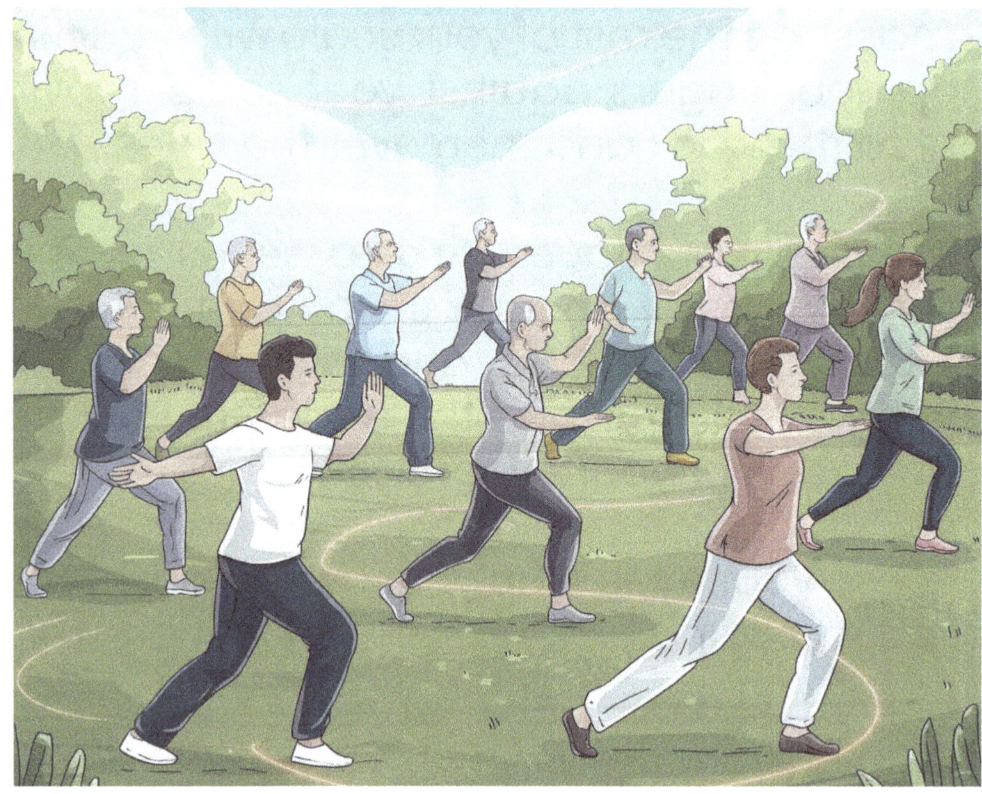

For maximum stress relief, add mindfulness to your workout While simply engaging in rhythmic exercise will help you relieve stress, adding a mindfulness component can benefit you even more.

As with meditation, mindful exercise requires being fully engaged in the present moment, paying attention to how your body feels right now, rather than your daily worries or concerns. Instead of zoning out or staring at a TV as you exercise, focus on the sensations in your limbs and how your breathing complements your movement.

If you're walking or running, **for example**, focus on the sensation of your feet touching the ground, the rhythm of your breath, and the feeling of the wind against your face. If you're resistance training, focus on coordinating your breathing with your movements and pay attention to how your body feels as you raise and lower the weights. And when your mind wanders to other thoughts, gently return your focus to your breathing and movement.

TIPS TO IMPROVE SLEEP QUALITY

- **Tip 1: Keep in sync with your body's natural sleep-wake cycle**

Getting in sync with your body's natural sleep-wake cycle, or circadian rhythm, is one of the most important strategies for sleeping better. If you keep a regular sleep-wake schedule, you'll feel much more refreshed and energized than if you sleep the same number of hours at different times, even if you only alter your sleep schedule by an hour or two.

- **Tip 2: Control your exposure to light**

Melatonin is a naturally occurring hormone controlled by light exposure that helps regulate your sleep-wake cycle. Your brain secretes more melatonin when it's dark—making you sleepy—and less when it's light—making you more alert. However, many aspects of modern life can alter your body's production of melatonin, shift your circadian rhythm, and make it harder to sleep.

- ## **Tip 3: Be smart about what you eat and drink**

Your daytime eating habits play a role in how well you sleep, especially in the hours before bedtime.

Focus on a heart-healthy diet. It's your overall eating patterns rather than specific foods that can make the biggest difference to your quality of sleep, as well as your overall health. Eating a Mediterranean-type diet rich in vegetables, fruit, and healthy fats—and limited amounts of red meat—may help you to fall asleep faster and stay asleep for longer.

Limit caffeine and nicotine. You might be surprised to know that caffeine can cause sleep problems up to ten to 12 hours after drinking it! Similarly, smoking is another stimulant that can disrupt your sleep, especially if you smoke close to bedtime.

Avoid big meals at night. Try to make dinnertime earlier in the evening, and avoid heavy, rich foods within two hours of bed. Spicy or acidic foods can cause stomach trouble and heartburn.

Avoid alcohol before bed. While a nightcap may help you relax, it interferes with your sleep cycle once you're out.

- **Can chair yoga be effective in managing chronic conditions?**

Yes! You can use chair yoga for seniors to reduce pain, increase mobility, and maintain physical function, helping to manage chronic conditions. Gentle movements and stretches can improve joint health and comfort. Yoga poses, breathing techniques, and meditation can all contribute to better mental health and emotional resilience, supporting seniors in having a positive perspective about their circumstances.

- **How does chair yoga improve balance and prevent falls?**

By strengthening the muscles used for stability, improving posture, and promoting better coordination, chair yoga can help with balance. Better balance can reduce the risk of falling, which is a major health concern for many seniors.

- **Can you lose weight or belly fat from doing chair yoga exercises for seniors?**

Any kind of yoga can support weight loss, including chair yoga! While it's not the most effective exercise for burning calories, it can support the mobility and functioning that keep you active, reduce stress that can lead to bad habits, make you more aware of your body, and facilitate habit change.

- **How long does it take to see results with chair yoga?**

The time it takes to see results from chair yoga will vary based on your unique circumstances, what you do, how often you practice, and what you're trying to achieve. Many clients start noticing changes within a few weeks or months.

- **How many times a week should you do chair yoga?**

Practicing chair yoga for seniors three times a week, or about every other day, is great! But any amount of yoga is useful, especially if you keep at it consistently over time.

- ## Which is better for seniors, Pilates or yoga?

While Pilates and yoga can both be beneficial to seniors, chair yoga is a great entry point that requires less skill to get started. If you're looking for group classes, it may be easier to find a yoga instructor with the knowledge and skills necessary to help you. If you're open to trying yoga therapy, it gives you the option to address specific pathologies, better manage pain, and improve mental and emotional health in addition to physical health.

- ## Where can I find chair yoga for seniors near me?

First, decide if you're looking for yoga therapy or group yoga classes. To find chair yoga classes for seniors near you, check local community centers, senior centers, gyms, or wellness clinics. If you're looking for a reputable yoga therapist, the International Association of Yoga Therapists has a database of certified yoga therapists. For those who would prefer to get guidance online, you can find yoga classes or yoga therapists to walk you through techniques from the comfort of your own home. This can also be helpful if you are struggling to find a suitable class or yoga therapist where you live.

Bonus Material

INSPIRATIONAL QUOTES TO KEEP YOU MOTIVATED

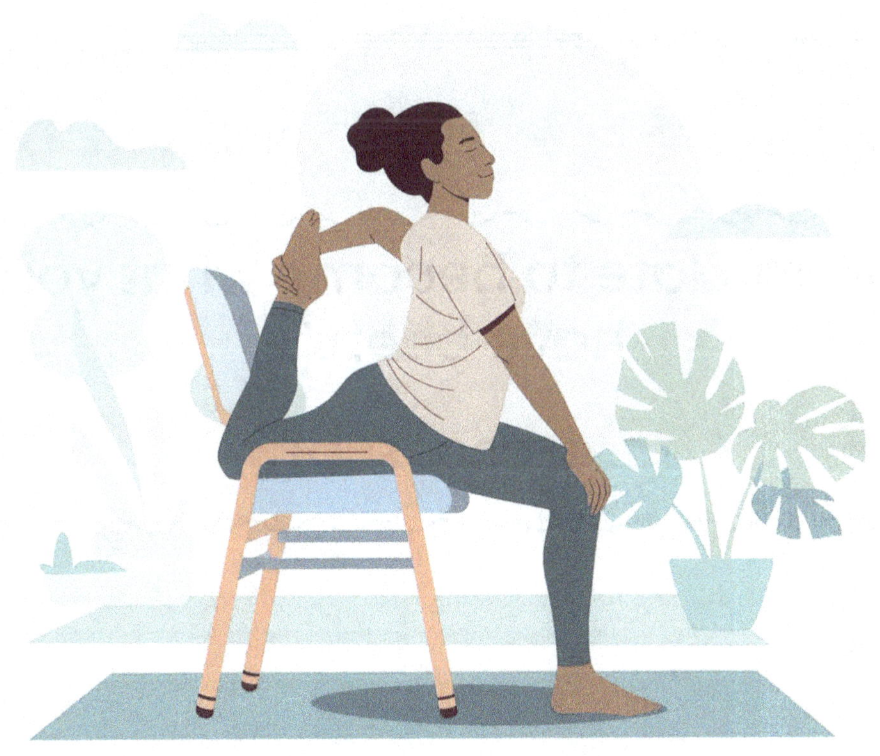

"Take care of your body. It's the only place
you have to live."

-JIM ROHN

"A healthy outside starts from the inside."

— ROBERT URICH

"It's never too late to become what you might
have been."

— GEORGE ELIOT

"Age is no barrier. It's a limitation you put on your mind."

– JACKIE JOYNER-KERSEE

"The first wealth is health."

– RALPH WALDO EMERSON

"It is exercise alone that supports the spirits and keeps the mind in vigor."

– MARCUS TULLIUS CICERO

"You don't have to be great to start, but you have to start to be great."

– ZIG ZIGLAR

"You're never too old to set another goal or to dream a new dream."

– C.S. LEWIS

"Exercise is king, nutrition is queen, put them together, and you've got a kingdom."

– JACK LALANNE